LIVING WITH FIBROMYALGIA

Fibromyalgia Symptoms & How to Live a Productive Life with Fibromyalgia through Diet and Exercise.

By **Lisa Gavit**

Living with Fibromyalgia

All rights reserved. This book may not be reproduced in whole or in part without written permission from the publisher, except by a reviewer who may quote brief passages in a review; nor may any part of this book be reproduced, stored in a retrieval system, or transmitted in any form or by any means, electronic, mechanical, photocopying, recording, or other, without written permission from the publisher.

Copyright © 2015 by Lisa Gavit

TABLE OF CONTENTS

Introduction

Causes of Fibromyalgia

Symptoms of Fibromyalgia

How is Fibromyalgia Diagnosed?

Fibromyalgia Treatments

Conclusion

Introduction

What is Fibromyalgia?

Fibromyalgia is a disorder characterized by widespread musculoskeletal pain accompanied by fatigue, sleep, memory and mood issues. Researchers believe that fibromyalgia amplifies painful sensations by affecting the way your brain processes pain signals.

Fibromyalgia can be a debilitating disorder. It that can strike at any time for those affected by it. The cause of fibromyalgia is unknown at this time but it is believed to involve psychological, genetic, neurological, and environmental factors. Fibromyalgia tends to affect women at a greater rate than men (about 9 women for every 1 man affected). It is believed fibromyalgia affects between 3-4% of the population. It has also been associated with rheumatoid arthritis, lupus, and as a side effect of anticholesterol medications.

Three to six million Americans have fibromyalgia, a long-term, muscle-effecting, pain-producing condition, and ninety percent of those who suffer with it are women. That is, 1 in every 73 people have the disease. Living with fibromyalgia can be like having a knot tied in your garden hose. Everything is flowing along normally, when suddenly, the flow of life slows down to a trickle and the joy dries up. Living with constant pain causes some to become prisoners in their

Living with Fibromyalgia

homes and even, their beds. Others drag themselves through daily routines with soreness and fatigue as constant companions. The intensity and area of symptom manifestation can vary with the weather, hormonal cycles, stress levels, and emotional states.

Living with almost constant pain can be a serious drain on a person's resources. Everyone knows what short term pain feels like, we have all hit our elbows on a hard surface, or stubbed our toes while walking barefoot, as bad as it hurts at least the pain finally goes away. For someone suffering from fibromyalgia, it may go away temporarily, and then return without any warning at all. Therapeutic massage, when performed properly, is a tremendous source of relief. It is a valuable tool that can help you maintain your sanity. There are a several things you can do to make life more bearable, the first of which is understanding your affliction

The complaints are always the same during a flare up, the muscles feel tight and ache severely, and the person starts to feel exhausted. To put a really tight muscle into perspective, think back about the last time you experienced a so called Charlie horse, the muscle tightened up for no reason and the pain was incredible. The reason most people don't understand, or for that matter, believe in fibromyalgia, is because it involves pain without trauma, yet everyone understands the pain of a Charlie horse, which by the way, always happens without any traumatic occurrence. Instinctively, when this happens, you do two things, stretch and rubbing the affected muscle, until it settles down and relaxes. The same approach should be used with your affliction. If the muscles are tight, you need to learn how to relax them. Those of you who have been suffering for years have no doubt learned by now that you cannot medicate your problem away. You have to try another approach if you want any type of lasting relief.

Relaxation techniques, along with therapeutic massage, are far better for your health compared to medicating yourself into oblivion. You should also understand that anxiety and emotional stress will trigger a flare up quicker than anything. Constant worry and despair can pretty much guarantee that you will not be able to find relief, so you will also have to learn how to control your emotions. A lot of people can trace the start of their pain back to some traumatic event in their life. It could be anything from being molested in your youth, to a bad marriage or child birth, the loss of a loved one, or some type of horrific accident. Whatever it might have been, you need to come to terms with it and put it behind you. Know this, the pain you are feeling is real, you are not imagining it, but the only way to conquer it is to go after the cause. There is no silver bullet or magic pill that will make it go away. The only way to resume a normal life is to attack it from every direction, using all the tools. Before being diagnosed, sufferers often fear they have something life-threatening wrong with them that no one can find or fix.

Living with Fibromyalgia

Causes of Fibromyalgia

As with any health problem that's not fully understood, there's lots of speculation about what causes Fibromyalgia.

This is a pretty complicated list, and obviously it's still a work in progress.

In general, though, the basic idea is that there's probably something that affects our physical and psychological perceptions of pain.

Some of these theories include:

Bodily tissues' inability to produce energy: Cells might be metabolically "shut down," leading to muscle pain and symptoms of fatigue.

Central nervous system abnormalities: Congenital malformations of the brain may disrupt the blood-brain barrier, potentially changing how the brain functions and responds to pain. In this case, viruses, stress, cell signal problems, pharmaceuticals, and nutrient deficiencies might act as triggers.

Altered sensory response in the brain: Some brain areas that process pain may be over-active, sounding the alarm without a legitimate threat.

Sleep deficiency: Short or poor-quality sleep can change hormone levels and immune function, increasing pain.

Inflammatory-pathway abnormalities: Cytokines, compounds that regulate how our immune system responds to inflammation, may be out of whack, causing a trigger-happy immune response to your body's own cells.

Too much stress: Allostatic load, or all of the stuff in your life that causes stress (workouts, kids, relationships, job, and so forth) might increase our pain perception.

Poor gut health: An imbalance of gastrointestinal bacteria (caused by an unhealthy diet or food intolerances) can lead to or worsen fibromyalgia symptoms including pain, fatigue and stress.

Use of antibiotics: There has been speculation that using antibiotics (or at least certain types at certain times) might contribute to the development of fibromyalgia by throwing gut bacteria off balance.

Hormone imbalances: Hormones particularly from the thyroid that are disrupted may cause hypersensitivity in the central nervous system, leading to the pain of fibromyalgia.

Pain-perception disorder: There may be an overproduction of pain-generating substances after injury (or even intense exercise).

Nutritional deficiency or toxicity: Pain may be triggered by deficiencies of B vitamins, vitamin C, and iron. And high levels of oxidative stress might play a role in the development of fibromyalgia (making dietary antioxidants important). Also, it might be worthwhile to check for candida overgrowth excessive levels of yeast in the gut caused by corticosteroid use, eating too many refined carbohydrates, or taking antibiotics.

Breathing disorders: Altered breathing (caused by problems like asthma and allergies) might cause an oxygen deficit, throwing blood gases out of balance. This could mess with the brain's processing of messages from pain receptors, leading to a fibromyalgia flare-up.

Infection: Getting sick (for example, with a virus) might initially trigger fibromyalgia.

A traumatic event: Adults with fibromyalgia report higher rates of childhood distress (e.g., maltreatment and abuse). Trauma might lead to fibromyalgia by causing endocrine disturbances or changes in the inflammatory system.

Environmental toxins: Chemicals you come into contact with can cause fatigue, headaches, chronic pain and other fibromyalgia symptoms.

Where you live: Adults in the United States may be more than twice as likely to develop Fibromyalgia compared to the global average. In China, for example, incidence of Fibromyalgia is minimal, perhaps because of genetic differences or sociocultural norms that affect the perception and acceptance of pain.

Living with Fibromyalgia

Unlike, say, smallpox or lead poisoning, where you can clearly blame a specific disease on a particular, clearly recognizable pathogen or toxin, there's no yet a smoking gun for Fibromyalgia.

Symptoms of Fibromyalgia

Fibromyalgia is a syndrome with many symptoms. Each individual with Fibromyalgia will have some of the symptoms. A few people will have all of the symptoms, but not everyone with Fibro has the same symptoms or even has symptoms all of the time. Also, symptoms may vary from day to day, year to year, or even minute to minute for each person coping with Fibromyalgia and other common coexisting conditions as well.

How confusing is that? Well, it gets even more confusing! Fibromyalgia patients have reported more than 200 symptoms. This comprehensive list of Fibromyalgia symptoms may actually be symptoms of other conditions that happen to commonly coexist with Fibromyalgia or they may be something that only one person experienced. Some of these symptoms are related and may in fact be different ways of describing the same symptom from different perspectives.

Living with Fibromyalgia

GENERAL

1) Activity level decreased to less than 50% of pre-illness activity level

2) Cold hands and feet (extremities)

3) Cough

4) Craving carbohydrates

5) Delayed reaction to physical activity or stressful events

6) Dryness of eyes and/or mouth

7) Edema

8) Fatigue, made worse by physical exertion or stress

9) Feeling cold often

10) Feeling hot often

11) Frequent sighing

12) Heart palpitations

13) Hoarseness

14) Hypoglycemia (blood sugar falls or low)

15) Increased thirst

16) Low blood pressure (below 110/70)

17) Low body temperature (below 97.6)

18) Low-grade fevers

19) Night sweats

20) Noisy joints with or without pain

21) Profuse sweating

22) Recurrent flu-like illness

23) Shortness of breath with little or no exertion

Living with Fibromyalgia

24) Severe nasal allergies (new or worsening allergies)

25) Sore throat

26) Sweats

27) Symptoms worsened by air travel

28) Symptoms worsened by stress

29) Tender or swollen lymph nodes, especially in neck and underarms

30) Tremor or trembling

PAIN

1) Abdominal wall pain

2) Burning Nerve Pain

3) Chest pain

4) Collarbone pain

5) Diffuse swelling

6) Elbow pain

7) Exacerbated Plantar arch or heel pain

8) "Growing" pains that don't go away once you are done growing

9) Headache – tension or migraine

10) Inflamed Rib Cartilage

Living with Fibromyalgia

NEUROLOGICAL

1) Blackouts
2) Brain fog
3) Carpal Tunnel
4) Feeling spaced out
5) Hallucinating smells
6) Inability to think clearly
7) Lightheadedness
8) Noise intolerance
9) Numbness or tingling sensations
10) Photophobia (sensitivity to light)

EQUILIBRIUM/PERCEPTION

1) Bumping into things
2) Clumsy Walking
3) Difficulty balancing
4) Difficulty judging distances (when driving, etc.)
5) Directional disorientation
6) Dropping things frequently
7) Feeling spatially disoriented
8) Frequent tripping or stumbling
9) Not seeing what you're looking at
10) Poor balance and coordination
11) Staggering gait

SLEEP

Living with Fibromyalgia

1) Alertness/energy best late at night
2) Altered sleep/wake schedule
3) Awakening frequently
4) Difficulty falling asleep
5) Difficulty staying asleep
6) Excessive sleeping
7) Extreme alertness or energy levels late at night
8) Falling asleep at random and sometimes dangerous moments
9) Fatigue
10) Light or broken sleep pattern

EYES/VISION

1) Blind spots in vision
2) Eye pain
3) Difficulty switching focus from one thing to another
4) Frequent changes in ability to see well
5) Night driving difficulty
6) Occasional Blurry vision
7) Poor night vision
8) Rapidly worsening vision
9) Vision changes

Living with Fibromyalgia

COGNITIVE

1) Becoming lost in familiar locations when driving
2) Confusion
3) Difficulty expressing ideas in words
4) Difficulty following conversation (especially if background noise present)
5) Difficulty following directions while driving
6) Difficulty following oral instructions
7) Difficulty following written instructions
8) Difficulty making decisions
9) Difficulty moving your mouth to speak
10) Difficulty paying attention
11) Impaired ability to concentrate
12) Inability to recognize familiar surroundings
13) Losing track in the middle of a task (remembering what to do next)
14) Losing your train of thought in the middle of a sentence
15) Loss of ability to distinguish some colors

Living with Fibromyalgia

EMOTIONAL

1) Abrupt and/or unpredictable mood swings
2) Anger outbursts
3) Anxiety or fear when there is no obvious cause
4) Attacks of uncontrollable rage
5) Decreased appetite
6) Depressed mood
7) Feeling helpless and/or hopeless
8) Fear of someone knocking on the door
9) Fear of telephone ringing
10) Feeling worthless
11) Heightened awareness of symptoms

GASTROINTESTINAL

1) Abdominal cramps
2) Bloating
3) Decreased appetite
4) Food cravings
5) Frequent constipation
6) Frequent diarrhea
7) Gerd-like Symptoms
8) Heartburn
9) Increased appetite
10) Intestinal gas
11) Weight gain
12) Weight loss

UROGENITAL

Living with Fibromyalgia

1) Decreased libido (sex drive)
2) Endometriosis
3) Frequent urination
4) Impotence
5) Menstrual problems
6) Painful urination or bladder pain
7) Pelvic pain
8) Prostate pain
9) Worsening of (or severe) premenstrual syndrome (PMS)

SENSITIVITIES

1) Alcohol intolerance
2) Allodynia (hypersensitive to touch)
3) Alteration of taste, smell, and/or hearing
4) Sensitivity to chemicals in cleaning products, perfumes, etc.
5) Sensitivities to foods
6) Sensitivity to light
7) Sensitivity to mold
8) Sensitivity to noise
9) Sensitivity to odors
10) Sensitivity to yeast (getting yeast infections frequently on skin, etc.)

Living with Fibromyalgia

SKIN

1) Able to "write" on skin with finger
2) Bruising easily
3) Bumps and lumps
4) Eczema or psoriasis
5) Hot/dry skin
6) Ingrown hairs
7) Itchy/Irritable skin
8) Mottled skin
9) Rashes or sores
10) Scarring easily

HAIR/NAILS

1) Dull, listless hair
2) Heavy and splitting cuticles
3) Irritated nail beds
4) Nails that curve under
5) Pronounced nail ridges
6) Temporary hair loss

How Is Fibromyalgia Diagnosed?

Unfortunately, there is not a single test to confirm fibromyalgia. Patients are generally diagnosed when all other known diseases or syndromes are ruled out. It is called differential diagnosis when used in medicine. Fibromyalgia is believed to be under-diagnosed with only about 25 percent of the actual cases being diagnosed properly.

The most widely accepted set of classification criteria for research purposes was elaborated in 1990 by the Multicenter Criteria Committee of the American College of Rheumatology. These criteria, which are known informally as "the ACR 1990", define fibromyalgia according to the presence of the following criteria:

- A history of widespread pain lasting more than three months affecting all four quadrants of the body, i.e., both sides, and above and below the waist.

- Tender points-there are 18 designated possible tender points (although a person with the disorder may feel pain in other areas as well). Diagnosis is no longer based on the number of tender points.

Fibromyalgia Treatments

Let us now take a look at few methods which can be quite effective in helping you regulate your symptoms and live a better life. It is important to maintain a healthy balance between relaxation and activities. This will help you better control the fatigue and pain associated with fibromyalgia. Don't keep working till you are almost ready to collapse. Set up a schedule for your daily activities and keep some fixed time for resting in-between different activities at fixed intervals. Stick to the plan and don't get ahead of yourself by trying to sneak in additional activities to your regular tasks.

Many people with fibromyalgia experience a string of bad days when their symptoms flare up and they stay in pain all day long. This is followed sometimes by one or more 'good' days where their symptoms seem to subside and they feel better. It is a natural tendency to try to hurry up and do all the activities you missed during those painful days. This is a grave mistake.

What happens when you try to get the most out of a good day? You try to get all your chores done. You try and finish all your shopping, or catch up on cooking or whatever it is you were unable to do because of the pain. You keep on doing all the tasks until finally you crash. Then the next few days you may not even feel like getting out of bed. There must be a better way to manage your fibromyalgia symptoms and still live your life.

Living with Fibromyalgia

The first step to getting a balance between work and rest is start timing your activities. Invest in a stop watch. Before you begin an activity set the stopwatch to say 10 minutes and make sure when the stop watch hits the mark, you stop whatever it is you are doing and take rest. It is easy to get carried away and lose track of time once you start doing anything. By using a stop watch you will learn to pace your activities. Soon you will no longer need the stopwatch. You will develop a mental timer which will notify you every time you overdo any task.

Separate your tasks into groups and order them based on priority. Space out the really tiring tasks so you get enough rest in between.

Every 15 minutes or so, change the position or angle in which you are standing or sitting. This will prevent any muscle from tightening up. Once in every hour, get up and walk a few steps. Do some stretching to loosen up the tense muscles in your body. Stretch out your hands to both sides. Stretch out your legs. Flex your back a little. Do these exercises gently taking care you do not overstretch any muscle.

Take care of the foods you eat. Note down all the types of food you eat and find out which foods seem to make your symptoms worse. Avoid these foods completely. If you are on the heavier side, start to lose weight. Fibromyalgia pain symptoms are worse for overweight people compared to those with ideal weight. Talk to your doctor and draw up an ideal nutrition plan to help you lose fat without starving yourself. Fibromyalgia can seem a miserable condition but careful planning and treatment can help you live a normal life.

However, there are things that each individual can do to make living with fibromyalgia easier on themselves as well as on those whom they love.

A Healthy Diet

The food you eat will determine how well you will feel. If you feed your body processed, non-nourishing foods it will not be getting the nutrients it needs to help combat a draining, difficult condition. It's tempting to cater to yourself when you feel bad but chocolate and potato chips will not build a healthy body. Plus, the weight you gain from snacking on junk will cause more stress on already aching joints and muscles. Make a decision to fill your tank with premium fuel. You'd do it for your car if the dealer said it was necessary to avoid costly problems and repairs. When you food shop, avoid the aisles of the market and stick to the foods located along the walls. There you'll find your fruits, vegetables, meats, and dairy. Build your diet with the natural items, things containing no additives, artificial sugars, and unhealthy fats. It may likely be a lifestyle change for you but so is living with fibromyalgia. If it makes a difference in the quality of the life you lead, is it not worth trying?

Here are some tips in establishing an effective fibromyalgia diet:

Living with Fibromyalgia

- A good fibromyalgia diet should exclude alcoholic beverages and smoking; also, caffeine is known to have undesirable effects on the fragile nervous system of people with fibromyalgia and therefore, all products containing caffeine (coffee, tea, carbonated soda, cocoa and chocolate) should be excluded from the fibromyalgia diet.

- An appropriate fibromyalgia diet should contain less dairy products, especially those that contain high levels of fat; consider using soy replacements instead (soy milk, tofu).

- Consume less wheat products, as they are not well tolerated by people with fibromyalgia.

- Reduce the amount of sugar in your fibromyalgia diet.

- Stay away from food products that contain additives, colorants and preservatives.

- Avoid any kind of fried foods; consider eating more boiled and baked foods instead.

- Add more home-made meals in your fibromyalgia diet; consume more soups, as they are better tolerated by the stomach.

- Consume more liquids.

- Reduce the amount of salt and spices in your meals.

- Reduce the amount of meat in your fibromyalgia diet.

- Consume plenty of vegetables and fruits, as they are a vital source of vitamins and minerals.

- Consider taking mineral and vitamin supplements

Diet plays a major role in the development of fibromyalgia. When the patients consume too many junk foods, fast and processed foods which do not provide the body with proper nutrients, then the body becomes toxic and nutrient deficient. According to studies it is very common among fibromyalgia sufferers to have high levels of toxins and many nutrient deficiencies.

Calcium, magnesium, serotonin and vitamin D are just a few of the deficiencies. Vitamin D is obtained naturally from the sun, and it is essential for helping the body to absorb calcium, and also helps to fight anxiety and depression.

Serotonin is a natural hormone that also helps with depression, and helps the body and mind to relax and sleep well at night. It is obtained from foods such as pineapples, mangoes, kiwi fruit, broccoli, tomatoes, avocados, melons, mushrooms, walnuts, hazelnuts and hickory.

Magnesium and Calcium are muscle regulators that help to control the muscle expansions and contractions. When the body is deficient it can lead to muscle spasms and cramping, which is a common symptom of fibromyalgia. These minerals can be obtained naturally from blueberries, cherries, cantaloupe, dates, grapefruit, guava, artichokes, asparagus, beet root, Brussels sprouts, amaranth, Brazil nuts, cashews, chestnuts and hazelnuts.

Exercise Routine

Even though the body is already fatigued and does not need any more physical strain, it is still necessary to engage in a regular exercise routine. Working with a physiotherapist, a trained professional at the gym, or going for short walks on a daily basis can help to strengthen the muscles, which in turn will reduce the pain.

For most fibromyalgia sufferers, the word "exercise" stands for nightmare... "What do you mean I should be doing fibromyalgia exercises? It's hard enough to get out of bed in the morning, much less to do regular household duties or go to work!"

Many fibromyalgia sufferers feel so exhausted and are in so much pain, that they rarely even go out of the house. Shopping, gardening, and family activities give way to reading, sitting at the computer, and watching TV. This is really a sad situation... to be forced by your own body to give up doing things that you used to love to do because the fibromyalgia symptoms take over. You find yourself planning out every move you make, pacing yourself so you won't overdo and cause a fibromyalgia flare.

So, how can you overcome your fibromyalgia symptoms and take your life back?

Living with Fibromyalgia

The old school of thought by medical specialists was to have the patient avoid physical exertion and get plenty of rest. They couldn't have been more wrong!

Instead of accelerating the fibromyalgia symptoms and incapacitating the sufferer, fibromyalgia exercises, started gradually and done in moderation at a pace that doesn't stress the sufferer, can have some very positive effects on the body and the mind. Fibromyalgia exercises benefits include better, more relaxing sleep; reduced levels of stress and depression; increased energy and endurance; and weight control.

Whether you choose daily walks, swimming or another form of low-impact exercise, just moving your body with low-impact fibromyalgia exercises can reduce your pain. Fibromyalgia muscle stiffness can be exercised away by building healthy muscle tissue which is more flexible, stronger and can increase your range of motion and allow you to physically do more. Some forms of fibromyalgia exercises that have been shown to provide the greatest benefit are:

- Walking
- Swimming
- Yoga and Tai Chi
- Pilates
- Stretching

- Light weight and strength training

- Aerobic activities

- Working out and cardio

Your goal is to improve your health. So, do only what you feel comfortable doing. If something hurts... stop! Even walking may be difficult at first. You may only be able to go for a few minutes at a time. That's normal! Set small goals then increase them over time. Be sure to select activities that you enjoy! Consider using a gym that specializes in "fibromyalgia exercises" or working with a physical therapist. But before starting professionally run fibromyalgia exercises or starting a cardio program, discuss your intentions with your physician to be sure your overall health is up to the challenge.

Why do fibromyalgia exercises work to make you feel better?

Research has shown that low-impact fibromyalgia exercises help to restore the body's neurochemical balance, generating a positive emotional response. The heart rate slows down with regular exercise which reduces adrenaline associated with increased stress response. Fibromyalgia exercises also boost the levels of natural pain-fighting "endorphins" and helps to reduce another fibromyalgia symptom... anxiety.

Another physiological benefit of fibromyalgia exercises is the regulation of the body's serotonin levels. Neurotransmitters like serotonin, is believed by medical and scientific communities to play a vital role in maintaining positive moods and promoting restful, healing sleep. Levels of serotonin which are usually low in fibromyalgia sufferers, can be increased by the sufferer participating in some regular fibromyalgia exercises. However, it's generally wise to avoid activities and exercises which require you to be doing a lot of jumping up and down (high impact), like basketball, volleyball, and some forms of dancing.

A Summary Fibromyalgia Exercises;

- Consistency is the key.

- Start slowly and increase your workout to about 30 minutes per day.

- Take your time... pace yourself... don't let others push you beyond where you are comfortable.

Take steps to improve your overall health, take control of your weight and start a nutritional supplement program to heal your body from the inside-out.

Reduce Physical Labor

Even though there are many causes of fibromyalgia, it is often caused by strenuous physical labor. Thus reducing physical activity and labor can help the muscles to somewhat relax and recuperate.

This may often mean to take a medical leave of absence from work, or to find another job that is less physically demanding.

Foods to Avoid

Foods that are high in unhealthy fats, processed foods, and all junk foods should be avoided whenever possible. Caffeine and alcohol should be reduced as they can interfere with sleeping.

Plenty of Rest and Sleep

Last but not least, getting plenty of rest and sleep is also very important to help the mind and body cope with the illness. Not receiving the proper rest that the body needs can contribute not only to the emotional pain, but the physical pain as well.

Are you receiving the best treatment for your fibromyalgia? Learn how nature can relieve your symptoms of this debilitating disease.

Living with fibromyalgia can literally turn your world up-side down. It feels as if the life you once had is all but gone.

Laugh and Enjoy

Crying, whining, and fear of the future will not change your fibro symptoms for the better. But laughing just might. If you have to live with fibro, then live well. You could spend your life bemoaning the fates that brought fibro into your life or you can make a decision to live your life well in spite of it. Don't let fibro take your joy from you. It's not the end of your life. It's just another obstacle along the way. Life with fibromyalgia is a balancing game. You balance doing the things you really need to do with the things that make you happy. It's an experiment where daily you learn more about yourself, what drains you, and what renews you. Give yourself permission to smile, to rest, to play again. Dream dreams. Take up hobbies, make a bucket list and then slowly, follow your dreams. Learning to live life fully is learning to know yourself, accept yourself with all of your weaknesses and gifts, and then giving yourself permission to live and live well.

Nutritional Aids

A few small treatment trials show that the nutritional supplements below may be beneficial for reducing your fibromyalgia symptoms, but larger studies are really needed.

Magnesium/Malic Acid/B vitamin Complex: Malic acid is a key sugar that is broken down in the muscles to make energy. Both magnesium and the B vitamins (B1 and B6) are needed for this process. One small study showed that this combo of supplements reduced muscle pain in fibromyalgia patients.

Omega 3 Fatty Acids: These oils are often referred to as anti-oxidants. They neutralize chemical byproducts that might otherwise harm your cell membranes and interfere with their ability to function. The best formulas contain roughly 500 mg of EPA and 500 mg of DHA (both omega 3s). DHA makes up about 15 percent of your brain's gray matter and it is vital for protecting your brain cells. A small study indicates that 2,500 mg of EPA/DHA combined per day helps ease fibromyalgia pain. Other larger studies show this supplement reduces triglycerides, protects your cardiovascular system, and works as a mild anti-depressant.

Anti-oxidants (Vitamins E and C): These two vitamins work as anti-oxidants to protect your cells and one study in fibromyalgia patients showed that this combination reduced the symptoms.

Melatonin and Valerian: Melatonin is not a powerful hypnotic, but it can regulate your body's internal clock to improve the quality of your sleep. Valerian is an herb that does have sedating properties that may ease you into sleep.

5-HTP: This molecule is easily absorbed and readily enters the brain where it is converted into serotonin (must be avoid with medications that boost serotonin). Increasing brain serotonin is believed to improve mood, and if taken at night could help some people sleep.

Acetyl L-Carnitine: A small trial in fibromyalgia patients showed that 500 mg of Acetyl L-Carnitine taken three times a day helped ease the pain and fatiguing symptoms of this condition.

Conclusion

Fibromyalgia is a disease that affects not only the sufferer but also those around him or her. It is an often misunderstood disease that can create frustration. Understanding and managing the symptoms is the goal. Proper choices and therapy can allow fibromyalgia patients to live normal productive lives.

An appropriate diet is vital for maintaining both physical and mental balance and it can strengthen the immune system of the organism. A good fibromyalgia diet can be a very effective way of overcoming the symptoms of the disorder, normalizing and stimulating the activity of the body. Unhealthy lifestyle, stress, lack of sleep, smoking, the abuse of alcoholic beverages are all considered to be factors of risk in the development of fibromyalgia. By improving your lifestyle and by respecting an appropriate fibromyalgia diet, you will quickly feel improvements in your health. Also, an effective fibromyalgia diet can considerably ameliorate the symptoms of the disorder.

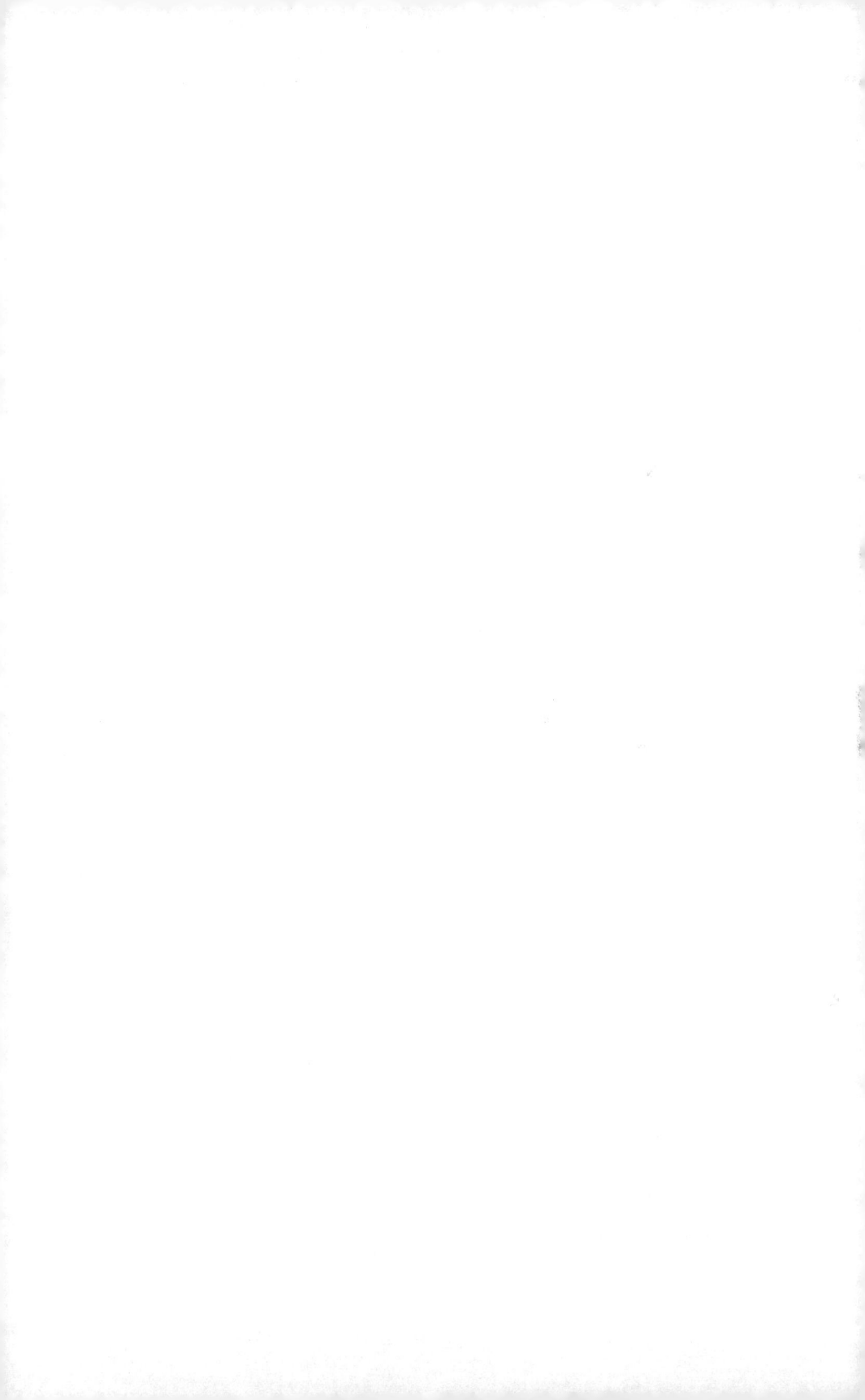

Printed in Great Britain
by Amazon